Dutch Oven Cooking the Scouting Way

"How to Make One-Pot Cast Iron Magic"

Dutch Oven Cooking the Scouting Way

"How to Make One-Pot Cast Iron Magic"

Compiled by Mike Matzinger

This is a compilation of Dutch oven recipes that are the favorites of Scouts in Troop 219 and Troop 600, Scouts BSA units based in Oak Ridge, NC. Cooking is a big part of the weekend outdoor adventures these troops experience every month. Now, you too can enjoy some of the great dishes these Scouts enjoy.

All profits from this compilation fund Troop 219 (The Sisterhood of Scouting).

Library of Congress Control Number: 2023946419

Cover design by Jasmine Mumford

Interior design by Jasmine Mumford and Brian Claspell

ISBN: 978-1-947315-14-3

ACKNOWLEDGMENTS

This cookbook wouldn't have been possible without thousands of Scouts who helped me develop and test a wide range of Dutch Oven recipes. In particular, thank you to the Scouts in Troop 219 for girls and Troop 600 for boys. These Scouts know how to cook amazing meals and aren't shy to trying new things.

I owe an enormous debt of gratitude to Anna and Brian Claspell who did the hard work behind the scenes in organizing the recipes. And, thank you to Brian and to Jasmine Mumford for design work.

A quality Scouting program doesn't happen on its own. Thank you to the following Assistant Scoutmasters who supported my Scouts in their development to become better versions of themselves – Kathy Bunthoff, Greg Ford, Nick Gee, James Gunter, Steve Holland, Ellen Mannella, Tim Nadeau, Richard Stanislawscky, Chris Sumner, Wyatt Wallace, and Sarah Wunner.

Lastly, thank you to the residents of the Northwest Guilford area for supporting Scouting. In particular, thank you to Northwest Guilford Woman's Club for sponsoring Troop 219 and Oak Ridge Presbyterian Church for sponsoring Troop 600.

Learn more about Scouting in the in North Carolina Northwest Guilford area:

Troop 219 www.troop219g.com

Troop 600 www.scoutdude.com

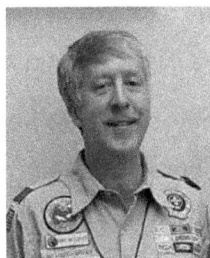

About the Author

Mike Matzinger has been involved in Scouting for almost 35 years, first as a youth participant and now as a volunteer at the local and national level. He and two of his sons are Eagle Scouts.

Mike has founded seven units in the Old North State Council, three of which he currently serves. He is Scoutmaster of 43 Scouts in Troop 219G and 71 Scouts in Troop 600B and he is Skipper of 18 Scouts in Ship 3. His focus is on providing the promises of Scouting to underserved communities including those with special needs.

Mike is the recipient of numerous Scouting awards including the Sea Scout Leadership Award, Venturing Leadership Award, Special Needs Scouting Service Award, Silver Beaver, and National Eagle Scout Association Outstanding Eagle Scout Award (NOESA). When not engaged in Scouting activities, Mike works as President of Burlington Chemical Company and serves Black Suit Initiative as Board Chair, Lionheart Academy as Board Member, and the International Federation of Scouting Rotarians as Area 7690 Coordinator.

Mike is married to Beth Matzinger. They have six children and are celebrating their first grandchild this fall.

CONTENTS

SECTION 1 – BREAKFAST

Bacon Quiche

Ingredients

1 pound package bacon
1 green bell pepper
1 onion
1 deep dish pie shell
3 cups shredded cheddar
6 eggs
¾ cup sour cream
5 ounces frozen chopped spinach

Instructions

Cook bacon in Dutch oven with chopped onion and chopped bell pepper until onion is translucent. Remove and set aside. Place pie crust into bottom of Dutch oven. Bake crust 5 minutes. Place bacon mixture into crust followed by cheese. In a small bowl, mix eggs, sour cream, spinach, salt, and pepper. Pour into pie shell. Bake covered until center is set.

Banana-Pecan French Toast

Ingredients

1 1/2 cups packed brown sugar

1 ½ sticks butter

1 cup chopped pecans (pea-cans)

1 cup pancake syrup

3 bananas

1 loaf cinnamon bread or day old French baguette

8 eggs

1 3/4 cups milk

1 teaspoon cinnamon

¼ teaspoon nutmeg

2 teaspoon vanilla extract

powdered sugar

Instructions

Mix in a bowl brown sugar, butter, pecans, and syrup. Gently stir in bananas. Spoon mixture evenly into a hot Dutch oven. Place 2 layers of bread over banana mixture, tearing bread slices to fit, if necessary. Beat eggs, milk, cinnamon, nutmeg, and vanilla extract and pour over bread. Allow to set 30 minutes. Bake until eggs are firm. Serve portions upside down, spooning sauce from bottom of dish over each serving. Sprinkle with powdered sugar.

Biscuits and Gravy

Ingredients

1-16 ounce can jumbo buttermilk biscuits
2 pounds sausage
1 cup flour
3 cups milk

Instructions

Place biscuits into greased and preheated Dutch oven and cook until golden brown. Remove biscuits and set aside. Cook sausage and then stir in flour. Slowly add milk and cook until mixture comes to a boil and thickens, stirring constantly. Season to taste with salt and pepper. Serve sausage gravy over biscuits.

Breakfast Burritos

Ingredients

1 pound bacon
1 pound sausage
1 onion
2 pounds frozen hash browns
12 eggs
12 large flour tortillas
1 pound shredded cheese
1 bottle ranch dressing
1 jar salsa

Instructions

Cook bacon, sausage, and chopped onion in Dutch oven until onion is translucent. Remove and set aside. Add hash browns to bacon grease and cook 30 minutes. In a bowl, beat eggs. Pour eggs and meat mixture over hash browns and cook covered until eggs are set. To serve, place several spoonful's on a tortilla, add cheese, ranch dressing, and salsa, and then roll up.

Deep Dish Breakfast Pizza

Ingredients

6 strips of bacon
½ pound breakfast sausage
1 clove garlic
1 teaspoon Italian seasoning
½ green bell pepper
½ red bell pepper
½ onion
5 mushrooms
6 eggs
1 tube refrigerator crescent rolls
2 cups shredded cheddar cheese

Instructions

Cook bacon in Dutch oven and remove. Brown sausage, drain grease, and mix in minced garlic, Italian seasoning, chopped peppers, chopped onion, and sliced mushrooms. Sauté 5 minutes. Stir in crumbled bacon. Remove mixture and set aside. Line Dutch oven bottom with unrolled crescent rolls creating a pizza crust by pinching the dough vertically along the sides up to 1 inch. Fill crust with mixture, pour in eggs, and sprinkle cheese on top. Cook covered until eggs are set in the middle.

Eggs Benedict Casserole

Ingredients

1 package sliced ham
1 onion
1 12 ounce package English muffins
12 eggs
3 cups milk
1 teaspoon mustard
2 teaspoon salt
1 teaspoon black pepper
packaged Hollandaise sauce

Instructions

Cook sliced ham with chopped onion in Dutch oven until onion is translucent. Add English muffins cut into 1 inch pieces. Mix eggs, milk, mustard, salt, and pepper and pour over Dutch oven mixture. Allow to rest 30 minutes. Then, cook covered until eggs set. Serve topped with Hollandaise sauce.

Mountain Man Breakfast

Ingredients

2 pounds bacon (or sausage)
1 onion
1 red bell pepper
1 green bell pepper
2 pounds frozen hash brown potatoes
18 eggs
2 pounds grated cheddar cheese

Instructions

Cut bacon into small pieces and cook with chopped onion and chopped peppers in Dutch oven until onion is translucent. Remove mixture and cook potatoes in bacon grease until golden brown. Add bacon mixture back to Dutch oven followed by beaten eggs. Cover and cook until eggs are almost solid. Sprinkle with cheese and continue cooking covered until eggs are set and cheese melted.

Sausage and Eggs Over Cheesy Grits

Ingredients

2 pounds sausage

1 onion

1 red bell pepper

12 eggs

3 cups Old Mill of Guilford grits

1 cup shredded sharp cheddar cheese

Instructions

Cook sausage, chopped onion, and chopped pepper in Dutch oven. Remove and set aside. In a pot, cook grits then add cheese and salt and pepper to taste. In Dutch oven, cook eggs sunny side up. To serve, top grits with sausage mixture and then place an egg on top.

Southwestern Omelet

Ingredients

12 strips of bacon
1 onion
1 jalapeno pepper
10 eggs
1 avocado
2 tomatoes
2 cups sharp cheddar cheese
1 jar salsa

Instructions

In Dutch oven, cook bacon, chopped onion, and minced pepper in oil and remove when onion is translucent. Pour beaten eggs into Dutch oven and cook 5 minutes. Combine onion, pepper, and bacon mix with chopped avocado, chopped tomatoes, and half the cheese. Spread over eggs and fold eggs over. Sprinkle remaining cheese on top and cook until melted. Top with salsa.

SECTION 2 – DINNER

Bacon Buffalo Mac and Cheese

Ingredients

- 1 pound medium shell pasta
- 2 (8 oz.) cream cheese
- 3 cloves garlic
- 2 cups wing sauce
- 2 cups ranch dressing
- 10 strips bacon
- 1 red bell pepper
- 4 cups Cheddar Jack cheese
- 2 cups break crumbs

Instructions

Cook pasta until done, then drain. In a bowl, lightly mix cream cheese (softened and cut into small squares), minced garlic, wing sauce, and ranch dressing. Cook bacon cut into 1 inch pieces. Add cooked pasta and pepper. Stir well to combine. Add cream cheese mixture and sprinkle bread crumbs. Cook covered until golden and bubbly, typically 30 minutes.

Bacon Cheeseburger Meatloaf

Ingredients

3 pounds ground beef

1 envelop onion soup mix

1 onion

6 cups shredded cheddar cheese

5 eggs

4 packets plain oatmeal

12 strips bacon

1 bottle barbeque sauce

Instructions

In a bowl, mix meat, soup mix, chopped onion, half the cheese, eggs, oatmeal, and one cup water. Press into Dutch oven, lay strips of bacon on top, and coat with sauce. Cook covered 90 minutes. Place remainder of cheese on top and cook until melted.

Beef Stroganoff

Ingredients

3 pounds ground beef or stew meat
2 onions
10 tablespoons flour
2 teaspoons garlic powder
1 teaspoon paprika
1/2 cup brown sugar
1 pound mushrooms
2 cans cream chicken soup
3 tablespoons Worcestershire sauce
2 tablespoons Dijon mustard
2 pints sour cream
2 12-ounce packages of egg noodles
1 stick butter

Instructions

Brown meat and sauté chopped onions in Dutch oven. Remove grease and stir in 4 tablespoons of flour. Add remaining ingredients except sour cream and noodles - chop onions and mushrooms before adding. Cook covered 30 minutes. Meanwhile, cook noodles as directed (not in the Dutch Oven). Stroganoff sauce is done when liquid approaches being pasty. If stroganoff sauce is thin, stir in remaining flour and cook 10 minutes longer. Then, stir in the sour cream. Salt to taste. Drain noodles, stir in butter, and add to sauce.

Cheeseburger Pie

Ingredients

3 pounds ground beef
2 onions
1 green bell pepper
2 cups shredded cheddar cheese
1 can diced tomatoes
2 cups Bisquick
1 cup milk
3 eggs

Instructions

In Dutch Oven, cook ground beef, chopped onions, and chopped pepper until onions are translucent. Remove grease and add tomatoes. In a mixing bowl, blend Bisquick, milk, and eggs. Pour Bisquick mix on top; do not stir in. Sprinkle cheese on top; do not stir in. Bake until knife inserted in center of Bisquick mixture comes out clean.

Chicken and Cheese Doritos Casserole

Ingredients

3 chicken breasts
2 packets taco seasoning
1 can black beans
2 cans kernel corn
1 can mild RO-TEL
1 tub sour cream
2 cans cream of mushroom soup
2 cans cream of chicken soup
4 cups Mexican blend cheese
1 bag Nacho Cheese Doritos, family size
1 container of cherry tomatoes
1 jar salsa
freshly chopped cilantro

Instructions

In a heated and oiled Dutch oven, cook chicken breasts cut up into small cubes and coated with both packets of taco seasoning. Add drained beans, drained corn, RO-TEL (not drained), half the sour cream, and cans of soup. Stir until cream cheese has melted. Remove chicken mixture from Dutch oven. Place a third of a bag on crushed Doritos on bottom of Dutch oven and spoon half of chicken mixture evenly on top followed by half of shredded cheese. Add another layer of Doritos (1/3 of the bag), then remaining chicken mixture, followed by remaining shredded cheese. Cook covered 30 minutes or until hot and bubbling. Add remaining crushed Doritos on top. Top with cherry tomato halves, salsa, sour cream, and cilantro when serving.

Chicken and Cashews

Ingredients

1 onion
1 green bell pepper
3 pounds boneless chicken breasts
3 carrots
4 stalks celery
2 cups cashew halves
1 cup sugar
½ cup vinegar
3 tablespoons ketchup
4 tablespoons cornstarch
1 can pineapple chunks
3 cups uncooked rice

Instructions

Place chopped onion and chopped bell pepper in pre-heated Dutch oven and Sauté in oil. Add chicken breasts cut into chunks, diced carrots, diced celery, and cashews. Simmer 15 minutes, stirring often. Add water, if needed. In a bowl, mix ½ cup water with sugar, vinegar, ketchup and cornstarch. Blend until smooth then stir in pineapple (including juice). Add pineapple mixture and cornstarch. Bring to a boil, stirring constantly. In a pot, prepare rice. Simmer 30 minutes or until chicken is done. Serve over hot rice.

Chicken and Rice

Ingredients

2 cups rice

1 chicken

1 packet dry onion soup mix

2 cans chicken broth

1 can cream of mushroom soup

3 stalks of celery

Instructions

Place uncooked rice in cold Dutch oven. Place cut up chicken parts on top of rice. Sprinkle dry soup mix on chicken. Add broth, soup, chopped celery, and 1 cup water. Cook covered 90 minutes.

Chicken Pasta

Ingredients

12 oz pasta
1 stick butter
1 onion
4 boneless chicken breasts
1 packet Italian dressing mix
1 jar pasta sauce
3 cups shredded cheese

Instructions

Boil pasta for half the recommended time to partially cook it. Rinse with cold water and set aside. Into hot Dutch oven add butter, chopped onion, and chicken cut up into chunks. After a few minutes, stir in Italian dressing mix. When chicken is nearly cooked, add pasta sauce, salt, and pepper. Simmer 5 minutes. Mix in half-cooked pasta and cheese. Cook 15 minutes or until pasta is soft.

Cowboy Beans

Ingredients

8 slices of bacon

1 onion

1 can baked beans

1 can kidney beans

1 can Lima beans

1/2 cup ketchup

1/3 cup packed brown sugar

2 teaspoon mustard

2 teaspoon cider vinegar

1/4 teaspoon salt

1 package Kielbasa

Instructions

Cook bacon, sliced into one inch segments, and chopped onion in Dutch oven until onion is translucent. In a bowl, combine beans, ketchup, brown sugar, mustard, vinegar, and salt. Add bean mixture to Dutch oven and simmer 20 minutes covered. Add sausage cut into 1 inch pieces and simmer for an additional 20 minutes uncovered.

Cranberry Chicken with Wild Rice

Ingredients

6 chicken breasts
1 package fast-cooking wild rice blend
2 butternut squash
1 jar cranberry sauce
2 tablespoons lemon juice
2 tablespoons soy sauce
2 tablespoons Worcestershire sauce
1 cup dried cranberries

Instructions

Place chicken in cold Dutch oven. In a bowl, mix 3 cups hot water with rice mix and pour over rice. Place chopped butternut squash around chicken. In a bowl, mix cranberry sauce, lemon juice, soy sauce, and Worcestershire sauce. Pour over chicken. Cook covered 1 hour. Top with dried cranberries.

Jambalaya

Ingredients

1 pound smoked sausage
1 large onion
1 green bell pepper
3 stalks celery
1 teaspoon Cajun seasoning
1 cup uncooked white rice
1 can diced tomatoes
1 tablespoon minced garlic
2 cups chicken broth
3 bay leaves
¼ teaspoon dried thyme
1 pound peeled and deveined shrimp

Instructions

Cook sausage, cut into one inch long pieces, in Dutch oven for 5 minutes and then add chopped onion, chopped pepper, chopped celery, and Cajun seasoning. When vegetables are soft, typically 10 minutes, stir in rice until evenly coated in the vegetable mixture, then pour in the tomatoes with juice, garlic, broth, bay leaves, and thyme. Simmer covered 20 minutes. After 20 minutes, stir in shrimp, and cook 10 minutes uncovered until shrimp turn pink and are no longer translucent in the center. Do NOT overcook. Discard the bay leaves before serving.

Lasagna

Ingredients

2 pounds ground beef
1 onion
2 large jars spaghetti sauce
2 teaspoons Italian seasoning blend
2 teaspoons garlic powder
1 tub ricotta cheese
1 tub cottage cheese, large curd
2 pounds shredded mozzarella cheese
3 eggs
1 pound lasagna noodles

Instructions

Cook meat and chopped onions in Dutch Oven until onion is translucent. Drain off grease. In a bowl, mix sauce, seasoning salt, and garlic powder. In another bowl, mix cheeses and eggs. Save ½ pound of mozzarella cheese for later. Line Dutch oven with foil and place a layer of noodles, break to fit. Spread 1/3 of meat mixture over noodles and ½ of cheese mixture over meat mixture. Break up additional noodles and place over top of preceding mixtures. Spread remaining meat mixture over noodles and remaining cheese mixture over meat mixture. Break up remaining noodles and place over cheese mixture. Spread remaining meat mixture over noodles. Pour three cups hot water between inside of Dutch oven and foil. Cook one hour or until noodles are soft.

Mexican Casserole

Ingredients

2 pounds ground beef
2 onions
2 packets taco seasoning
3 cans chili with beans
1 can whole kernel corn
1 can diced tomatoes
1 can crushed pineapple
1 can sliced black olives
8-oz package shredded cheddar cheese
3 boxes Jiffy corn muffin mix

Instructions

Sauté beef and chopped onions in Dutch Oven until onions are translucent. Remove grease. Stir in taco seasoning. Open cans, drain all liquids, and add all. Add cheese. Stir thoroughly. Salt and pepper to taste. Prepare bread mix according to directions on box. Spread mix on top; don't stir in. Cook until knife placed into the muffin mix comes out clean.

Patrol Chili

Ingredients

3 pounds ground beef, turkey, or sausage
1 green pepper
1 onion
2 cans crushed tomatoes
1 tablespoon garlic flakes
2 tablespoon chili powder
2 teaspoon salt
1/2 teaspoon oregano
1/2 teaspoon cumin
2 cans kidney beans
1 can whole kernel corn

Instructions

Cook meat, chopped green pepper, and chopped onion in Dutch Oven until onion is translucent. Drain off grease. Add remaining ingredients except corn and beans. Simmer uncovered 30 minutes. Stir in undrained beans and corn. Simmer an additional 30 minutes uncovered. Serve with blackened corn bread.

Patrol Stew

Ingredients

2 pounds stew meat

2 onions

1 jar tomato paste

4 potatoes

1 cup baby carrots

1 cup mushrooms

1 bag mixed vegetables

1 packet beef stew seasoning mix

1 teaspoon paprika

1 teaspoon Worcestershire sauce

2 bay leaves

2 beef bouillon cubes

2 cans mushroom soup

Instructions

Season meat with salt and pepper and brown in Dutch oven with oil and chopped onions. Add tomato paste and cook 10 minutes. Add cubed potatoes, baby carrots, sliced mushrooms, mixed vegetables, seasoning mix, paprika, Worcestershire sauce, bay leaves, bouillon cubes, and soup. Cook covered 2 hours, then uncovered 1 hour. Thicken with cornstarch, if necessary. Remove bay leaves prior to serving.

Pork Chops and Potatoes

Ingredients

4 pork chops
1 stick butter
3 cups seasoned bread crumbs
3 potatoes
2 onions
1 can cream of mushroom soup

Instructions

Season pork chops with salt and pepper and add to heated Dutch oven coated with oil. Brown on both sides. Melt butter in a separate pan and then mix with bread crumbs and 1 cup of water. Pour mixture over pork chops. Place potatoes slices and chopped onions on top of pork chops and then cover with soup and ½ cup water. Cook covered 1 hour or until potatoes are tender.

Pot Roast

Ingredients

6 pounds chuck roast
3/4 cup flour
1 packet dry onion soup mix
1 cup ketchup
1 bag baby carrots
4 potatoes
1 onion
3 garlic cloves
2 bay leaves
2 cups beef stock

Instructions

Coat roast with flour and season with salt and pepper. Brown in hot Dutch oven with oil. Sear each side until well browned. Sprinkle on soup mix and add ketchup, baby carrots, potatoes cut into 2 inch pieces, chopped onion, cloves, and bay leaves. Cook covered 15 minutes and then add beef stock. Cook covered for 3 – 4 hours until meat is tender. Remove bay leaves prior to serving.

Pulled Barbeque Chicken Sandwiches

Ingredients

1 onion
2 garlic clove
2 teaspoon paprika
4 boneless chicken breasts
2 cups barbecue sauce
1 teaspoon hot sauce
½ cup chicken broth
12 hamburger buns

Instructions

Sauté chopped onion and minced garlic for 5 minutes in oil. Then, add paprika and chicken. Add 1 cup water and barbecue sauce, hot sauce, and broth. Simmer covered 60 minutes. Once chicken is tender, remove and shred with two forks. Bring sauce mixture to a boil until reduced to half in volume. Then, add shredded chicken back into Dutch oven and heat covered 10 minutes. Spoon chicken mixture on a bun.

Quartermaster's Stew

Ingredients

3 pounds hamburger meat or stew meat

1 onion

2 packets stew seasoning mix

2 cans mixed vegetables

2 cans potatoes

1 can chopped tomatoes

sliced mushrooms

Instructions

Cook meat and chopped onions in Dutch oven until onion is translucent. Drain off grease. Stir in seasoning mix and cook uncovered 15 minutes. Add vegetables (drain liquid before adding) and potatoes (do not drain). Cook 20 minutes uncovered. Add tomatoes and mushrooms (drain liquid before adding). Continue cooking uncovered until potatoes are tender.

Ravioli

Ingredients

1 (25 oz.) bag frozen sausage ravioli
1 large jar spaghetti sauce
1 cup Parmesan cheese
1 cup shredded mozzarella cheese

Instructions

Place thin layer of sauce on the bottom of Dutch oven followed by single layer of thawed ravioli. Cover ravioli with half of sauce. Sprinkle in half parmesan cheese. Place another layer of ravioli on top of sauce. Pour in rest of sauce. Top with mozzarella cheese and remaining Parmesan cheese. Cook covered 45 minutes. When done, sauce should be bubbling and cheese slightly brown.

Shepherd's Pie

Ingredients

2 pounds ground beef

2 onions

3 packets plain oatmeal

1 envelop onion soup mix

1 can tomato paste

1 can diced tomatoes

1 can peas

1 can sliced carrots

1 can kernel corn

2 packets garlic flavored instant potatoes

1 bag shredded cheddar cheese

Instructions

In Dutch oven, brown meat with chopped onions. Add 2 cups of water, oatmeal, soup mix, tomato paste, tomatoes, peas, carrots, and corn – drain liquid from all cans before adding. Prepare instant potatoes and cover. Cook covered 60 minutes. Place cheese on top and cook until melted.

Sloppy Joes

Ingredients

2 pounds ground turkey or beef
1 onion
1 green bell pepper
1 can crushed tomatoes
1/2 cup ketchup
2 tablespoons brown sugar
1 tablespoon white vinegar
1 tablespoon Worcestershire sauce
1 tablespoon steak sauce
½ teaspoon garlic salt
¼ teaspoon ground mustard
1/2 teaspoon paprika
2 tsp chili powder
8 to 10 hamburger buns, split

Instructions

In Dutch oven, cook beef, chopped onion, and chopped pepper until meat is no longer pink and the vegetables are tender. Drain grease. Stir in remaining ingredients and simmer 30 minutes. Spoon about ½ cup meat mixture onto each bun.

Tex Mex Creamy Chicken Casserole

Ingredients

- 1 stick salted butter
- 4 chicken breasts
- 1 packet taco seasoning
- 2 cans creamed corn
- 1 can black beans
- 2 cans diced tomatoes with green chilies (Ro-Tel)
- 3 cups Mexican style cheese blend
- 4 Tbsp. chopped fresh cilantro
- 1 jar salsa
- 1 tub sour cream
- 12 small tortillas

Instructions

Place butter and chicken breast pieces into heated Dutch oven. When chicken is no longer translucent, add taco seasoning. Remove chicken and mix in a bowl with corn, beans, tomatoes, 1 cup cheese, and cilantro. Layer 6 tortillas in bottom of Dutch oven. Top with half of chicken mixture. Repeat layer with remaining tortillas and chicken mixture. Simmer covered 30 minutes then sprinkle with remaining cheese and continue cooking until cheese has melted. Top with sour cream, salsa, and more cilantro, if desired.

SECTION 3 –DESSERTS

Apple Crisp

Ingredients

12 apples
3/4 cup lemon juice
1 cup sugar
1 cup raisins
2 tablespoons cinnamon
2 cups brown sugar
2 cups flour
1 tablespoon nutmeg
1 bag honey oat granola

Instructions

Place 12 peeled and sliced apples, lemon juice, sugar, and raisins in cold Dutch oven. Place on top a mixture of cinnamon, sugar, flour, nutmeg, and granola. Cook covered 30 minutes or until apples are tender.

Baked Stuffed Apples

Ingredients

10 baking apples
1 cup raisins
1 teaspoon cinnamon
1 teaspoon nutmeg
12 ounces orange juice concentrate
10 tablespoons honey
1 bag honey oat granola

Instructions

Remove core of apples but leave ½ inch of core on one side to form a cavity. In a bowl, prepare a filling by combining raisins, cinnamon, and nutmeg. Stuff each apple with filling. In a bowl, mix 3 cups water, juice concentrate, and honey. Place stuffed apples in hot Dutch oven and pour juice mixture over apples. Cook covered 1 hour or until apples are soft. Spoon excess sauce over apples and serve topped with granola.

Blueberry Buckle Cake

Ingredients

1 1/2 cups all-purpose flour
1/2 cup brown sugar
1 teaspoon ground cinnamon
1 stick butter
1 package white cake mix
1 package vanilla flavor instant pudding mix
4 cups blueberries

Instructions

Mix in bowl flour, sugar, and cinnamon. Mix in slices of butter until a crumbled texture is achieved. Prepare cake batter as directed on package (eggs and oil may be required). Add dry pudding mix. Add blueberries to hot Dutch oven and dump above two mixes on top. Cook covered 40 minutes or until knife inserted into cake comes out clean.

Chocolate Cherry Cobbler

Ingredients

2 sticks butter
1 large box chocolate cake mix
2 cans cherry pie filling

Instructions

Melt 1 stick butter in the bottom of Dutch oven. Add cherry pie filling. Add cake mix – prepare mix according to directions on box before adding (eggs and oil may be required). Cut 1 stick butter into patties and place on top. Cook covered 40 minutes or until knife inserted into cake comes out clean.

Dutch Oven Cheesecake

Ingredients

Graham cracker pie crust
5 packages (8 oz.) cream cheese
1 cup sugar
3 tablespoons flour
1 tablespoon vanilla
1 cup sour cream
4 eggs

Instructions

Place pie crust in hot Dutch oven and allow to warm 10 minutes. In a bowl, mix softened cream cheese, sugar, flour, and vanilla. Then mix in sour cream followed by eggs. Add eggs, one at a time, mixing until just blended. Cook covered 45 minutes or until center is almost set.

Peach Cobbler

Ingredients

2 sticks butter
1 large box yellow mix
2 cans peach pie filling

Instructions

Melt 1 stick butter in bottom of Dutch oven. Add peach pie filling. Add cake mix – prepare mix according to directions on box before adding (eggs and oil may be required). Cut 1 stick butter into 1 inch patties and place on top. Cook covered 40 minutes or until knife inserted into cake comes out clean.

Pineapple Upside Down Cake

Ingredients

2 sticks butter
1 cup brown sugar
1 can pineapple slices
1 can stemless cherries
1 box yellow cake mix

Instructions

Melt butter in the bottom of Dutch oven. Sprinkle brown sugar over butter and then arrange pineapple slices with a cherry in the center of each slice. Add prepared cake mix (check instructions on box to see if eggs and oil are required) with pineapple juice substituted in place of water. Cut 1 stick butter into 1 inch patties and add on top. Cook covered 40 minutes or until knife inserted into cake comes out clean.

Pumpkin Spice Pie

Ingredients

2 cans 100% pure pumpkin
2 tablespoons pumpkin pie spice
5 eggs
2 cups sugar
1 teaspoon salt
1 teaspoon cinnamon
2 teaspoons vanilla
3 cups evaporated milk
1 package yellow cake mix
2 cups chopped pecans
2 sticks butter

Instructions

In a bowl mix pumpkin, spice, eggs, sugar, salt, cinnamon, vanilla, and milk. Place mixture in hot Dutch oven. In a bowl mix cake mix, pecans, and butter and then sprinkle mixture on top. Cook covered 45 minutes or until knife placed in the pie comes out clean.

Seven Layer Brownies

Ingredients

1 box brownie mix
1 stick butter
1 tsp vanilla
1 cup toffee bits
1 cup semisweet chocolate chips
1 cup chopped pecans
1 cup small pretzels
½ cup + 2 tbsps. sweetened condensed milk

Instructions

In large bowl, blend brownie mix, melted butter, and vanilla. Place mixture into Dutch oven lined with foil. Cook covered 15 minutes. Sprinkle toffee bits, chocolate chip bits, and pecans (in that order) over partially cooked brownies. Drizzle with sweetened condensed milk to within 1 inch of sides. Sprinkle top with chopped pretzels. Cover and continue cooking for an additional 30 minutes or when knife inserted comes out almost clean. Do not over bake.

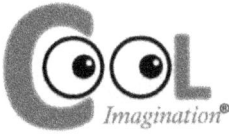

Cool Imagination Titles

Dutch Oven Cooking the Scouting Way
Compiled by Mike Matzinger

Enjoy a Dutch oven treat and support the next generation of servant leaders who are currently in scouts.

Convergence by Brian Claspell
Jim Conrad may not be as fictional as the CIA thinks. Pick up *Convergence*, a mystery-thriller, on Amazon and at other fine retailers.

One Spark - Short Story Winners and Finalist
Enjoy reading the short stories by talented young writers taken from the winners and finalists of the annual "Imagination Begins with You…" high school writing contest which was started in 2011. All proceeds support scholarships.

> ➤ *One Spark - Short Story Anthology 2011-2018*
> ➤ *One Spark – "Imagination Begins with You…" 2019*
> ➤ *One Spark – "Imagination Begins with You…" 2020*
> ➤ *One Spark – "Imagination Begins with You…" 2021*
> ➤ *One Spark – "Imagination Begins with You…" 2022*
> ➤ *One Spark – "Imagination Begins with You…" 2023*